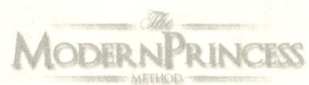

4 WEEKS TO A NEW YOU

Fitness and Weight loss is often equated with willpower and great discipline which in the past has made it almost impossible for you to reach and maintain your goals. With busy social lives, working, schooling are often surrounded with ample opportunities to make poor choices. Because disciple and willpower aren't our strongest points, I've created this 4 WEEK Fitness and Weight-loss Method to combine a little willpower, a little discipline and a lot of practicality to make it feasible for you to take on a new lifestyle. The goal is to lose inches, tighten your curves, build confidence and create an effortless approach to fitness and health as part of your ModernPrincess Lifestyle. With this method you will learn structure which indirectly channels discipline and you will learn to eat with sensuality keeping you from overeating. You will have flexible fitness options in your program so you can always feel on top of your game with options for lazy days, regular days and those days when you are just on fire.

As you prepare to start your 4 week Jump-Start Program get excited to welcome new changes on both the physical and metaphysical level. Your fourth week will be the most impressive, as you clearly see and feel the changes.

Initially, not everyone around you will be encouraging, as they won't understand what or why you are doing. Staying true to your morning routine (#princesstime) despite what kind of day you are initially experiencing will bring solitude, clarity and direction to your day and life.

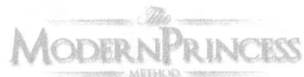
4 WEEK FITNESS AND WEIGHT-LOSS JUMP START PROGRAM

This JUMP-START Program is designed to give you a structured yet flexible and practical path in which you will be equipped with material to take drivers seat in your weight-loss and fitness regimen. Strict diets and exercise regimens make it easy to lose motivation causing you to binge and eventually repeat the cycle. With this method you will find pleasure in starting your day by taking care of yourself first. No matter what type of day you are experiencing, you can start and end it by being kind to yourself.

PART 1 #PRINCESSTIME

 DAILY MORNING ROUTINE:

Good Morning Princess. No matter where you are, what you did the night before, or how much weight you have to lose, you absolutely need to start your day on the right foot. Upon awaking, you are to brew yourself a cup of hot water and lemon or premium grade green tea. As you steep and cool your beverage, comfortably position yourself in front of a large mirror and begin your affirmations followed by visualization. This is called #princesstime, time to love yourself, it is all about you and only you.

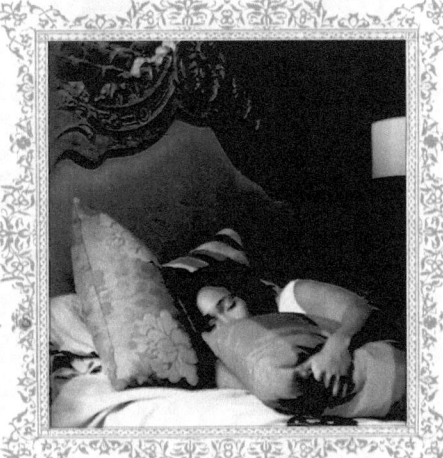

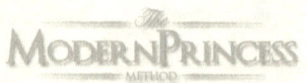

PART 1 #PRINCESSTIME

 AFFIRMATIONS:

Affirmations are the cornerstone of your #princesstime. These are words and phrases you say to yourself in present and first person in front of a mirror.The task is to affirm your desired outcomes. Example: I AM a thin eater, I AM beautiful, I AM organized, I AM capable, I AM patient, I AM lovable, I AM loving, I AM prosperous, I AM cheerful, I AM creative, I AM a diligent business woman, I AM goal setter, I AM a ModernPrincess, etc... Feeling your affirmations is what will make them powerful.

It is important that you state your affirmations as and how you would if your desired outcome were actually true. If you are experiencing difficulty with becoming one with your-I am's then ease into them by saying "I am thinner today than yesterday , I am becoming more and more energetic everyday or I am more and more lovable and loving everyday". The subconscious mind accepts whatever you feel to be true so if saying "I am thin" feels like a lie it therefore only reinforces that you are in fact "out of shape". Use the phrase that makes you feel the best so long is it in first person and in the now.

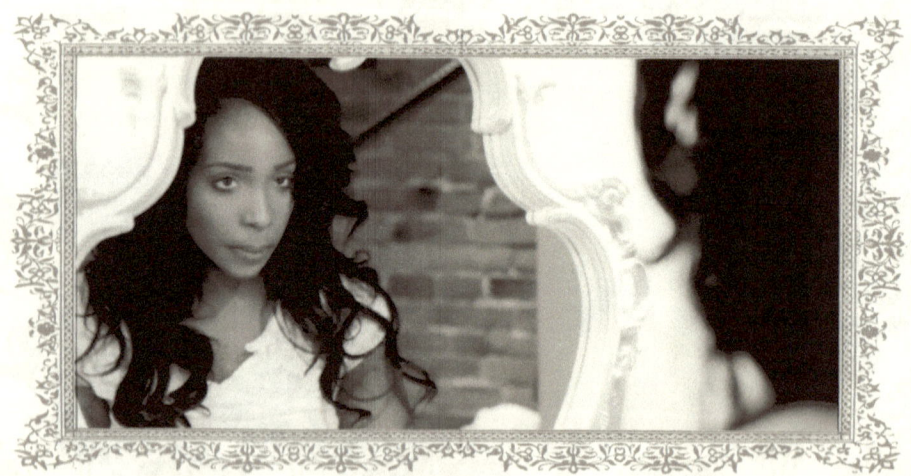

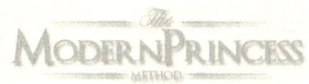
PART 3 #PRINCESSTIME

End your days by reviewing your diary and congratulate yourself in the choices you've made today. No day is a failure. Reinforce your "I AM's" during the last 20 minutes before sleep. By day 21, #princesstime will be part of you because self discovery and self improvement will be your daily goal. Waking up 15-45 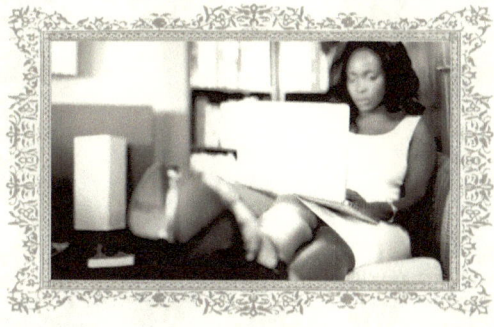 minutes earlier than usual, making and keeping to your to-do list, facing yourself and repeating words that might be uncomfortable at first, eating when you are truly hungry, eating slowly and stopping when you are satisfied will not be easy at first but stick to it and you will be pleased with yourself. By the end of 4 weeks, you will have learnt self-discipline, the basics of creating the life you want to live and you will have an increased regard for yourself. You are a ModernPrincess, wear it with pride. You created this! Day 30 is not the last day, it is the first day of which you can choose to be who so ever you wish to be by simply channeling your inner princess through your daily #princesstime.

To complete your journey, go to amodernprincess.com

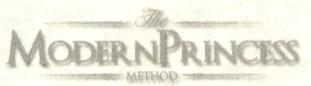

PART 2 #PRINCESSTIME

 ## VIGOR:

Vigor can be an intense full body workout set to get your heart pumping, burning fat with a dynamic cardio routine whilst tightening your trouble areas in 20 minutes or less. A great option is to pick 4 challenging exercises and perform them in 20 second intervals with 10 second rest periods. Example: 20 seconds of burpees, 10 seconds rest, 20 seconds of jump squats, 10 seconds of rest, 20 seconds of mountain climbers, 10 seconds of rest, 20 seconds of side kicks, 10 seconds of rest. Repeat. Perform 10+ days.

 ## POWER:

Most of your days should begin with "power" as this is the way you should be feeling on most mornings. Power can be a combination of interval training (such as Vigor) and weight-lifting. An average power workout should span 30-45minutesto ensure that you are heart pumping, butt toning, abs sculpting and melting stubborn fat. Perform 15+days.

PART 3 #PRINCESSTIME

 ## PRINCESS DIARY:

Now the fun part is done, its time to take on the world and the day with organization. Being organized and keeping a list of things to be completed today will keep you on track in all your goals. Take 5 minutes as you cool down after your workout to make a list of all the things you (A) must do (B) would like to do. If you choose to perform your exercise later in the day, simply follow your affirmations/ visualization with goal listing. As your day goes along, record your feelings, what you are eating and drinking and make a note of any achievements you may have discovered since changing your lifestyle. You may notice you had been losing valuable time or eating out of habit. You may notice little changes such as reaching for tea instead of soda, eating smaller meals and enjoying a calming walk at the end of the day.

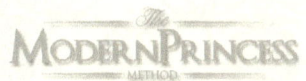

PART 2 #PRINCESSTIME

Now that you are eating like a thin eater, making healthy decisions, referring to yourself as the ModernPrincess you are transforming into and creating your very own enchanted life, do not be surprised when you notice that your days will start with an incredible amount of energy and excitement to take on the world. Following PART 1 of your morning routine you may energize your body's cells by using one of the three fitness regimens that I have created for you to combine toning and fat burning. If you haven't picked up the Modern-Princess Fitness DVD's, find other forms of exercise that suit you but remember to just do it. Regardless of the type of day you are experiencing, there is a sweat inducing workout for you to perform in the comfort of your home even 15 minutes makes a difference.

 TRANQUILITY:

PMS'ing, lost valuable sleep, hung-over or simply can't be bothered to jump around? Do not worry, a yoga and stretch combination will still be challenging yet a low key workout; all you need is a matt. It's on days when you don't feel like doing it is when you actually need it the most so take time to stretch out any kinks that may be causing you heavy tensions. On TRANQUILITY days, add a 20-30 minute walk after dinner. Perform 5-10 days.

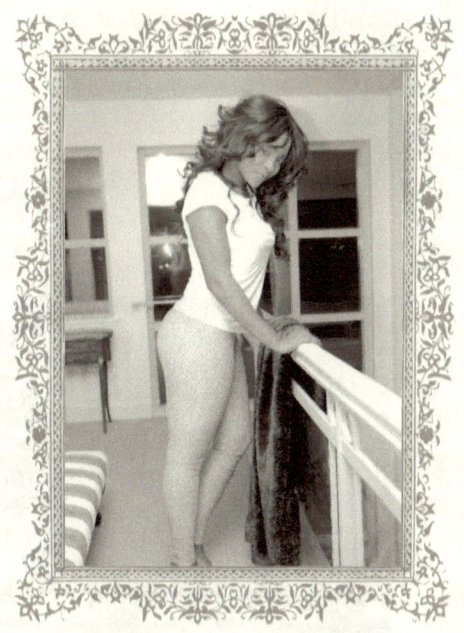

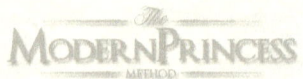

PART 1 #PRINCESSTIME

 VISUALIZATION:

There is a part of your brain that doesn't know the difference between real and imaginary activity. When you imagine or visualize things and experiences you want, that part of your brain begins to perceive them as reality. Visualizing allows you to feel the feelings you would feel if your desires where fulfilled. Along with feeling your affirmations, being in the now when visualizing is powerful in affirming your desires. Visualize your perfect body see how you would walk, speak, handle things and how others would speak of you. Visualize yourself eating slowly, choosing to eat vegetables and declining second helpings past the point of satisfaction. Also visualize how clothes would fit. As you do this, be IN the picture as a participator and not as an observer.

By starting your day on this note, you are becoming congruent with the ModernPrincess mindset; the proven mindset for success. Connecting to your inner princess will also bring to your life, absolute clarity about your life. You now know that it is within that you must go whenever you are needing guidance. Devote the first 15-45minutes of your day to yourself. No cell phone, no media, including but not limited to internet, radio and TV.

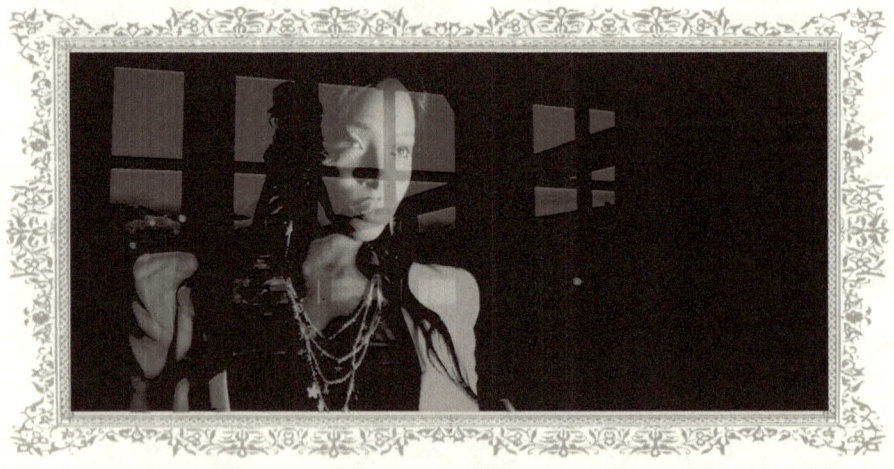

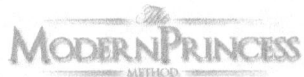

WEIGHT MANAGEMENT

 WEIGHT MANAGEMENT SIMPLIFIED:

*Wait for True Hunger - Just because it is lunch hour does not mean your body is calling for food. Wait for your body to tell you when it is truly hungry (not famished but moderately hungry). Drink 2-3 cups of stevia sweetened green tea or warm lemon water when the nagging desire to eat comes knocking before experiencing true hunger. You very well might be thirsty, not hungry.

*Eat Food You Truly Enjoy - If you eat something you don't like you will be left feeling unsatisfied and wanting what you really enjoy. When choosing your foods, remember that what you are looking to achieve is balance in all aspects of life so eat a balanced amount of carbohydrates, proteins and fats. Always pair any carbohydrates with protein. If you want the burger, have the burger but skip the fries etc...

*Eat Real Food - Most overweight people are overfed yet under nourished. If you aren't getting live nutrients to your body's cells, you are likely to be starving on a nutritional level thus keeping your body in the "starvation" mode. Your brain will continue to send hunger signals because although you are well fed on calories you could be underfed on nutrients. Add a salad or puree vegetable soup to your meals. Begin incorporating fresh pressed vegetable and fruit juices, nuts and fish to your diet whilst staying away from refined grains and deep fried foods.

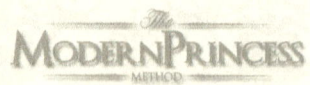
WEIGHT MANAGEMENT

 WEIGHT MANAGEMENT SIMPLIFIED (CONT):

*Eat Sensually - Make love to your food. Add just the right amount of salt, pepper, or any condiments and spices to your food, make every bite count, put your fork down and chew oh so slowly. Remember the texture, the crunch and the after taste. Yes it sounds silly but do it, it will change your life. You will begin to notice how certain foods just aren't as appetizing anymore.

*Hara Hachi Bu - Eat until you are 80% full. Stop eating when you begin to feel full. Now that you are eating slowly, you will notice how much less you will be eating. Don't ruin a good meal by a spoonful!

*Do Not Weigh Yourself - You may however measure your body around your arms, waist, chest, thighs, buttocks and calves. You may weigh yourself every 4-6 weeks but not everyday, doing so will drive you crazy. In the book ModernPrincess-A young woman's guide to living a balanced life-, I write about awareness. When you are aware, you are connected, you will know if you are feeling bloated, hungry, constipated, thirsty, tired or needing to detox.

*Actively Involved - Be actively involved in your fitness and well-being. Take the stairs, walk to work, stretch at the end of the day, practice good posture and before you eat, ask yourself, '"What do I really want?".

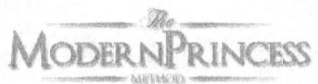

The
MODERN PRINCESS
METHOD

DAILY WEIGHT LOSS DIARY

TODAY'S DATE: _____

NUTRITION LOG:

BREAKFAST: DINNER:

LUNCH: SNACKS:

EXERCISE:

FITNESS:

MIND AND SPIRIT:

WAKE UP: TODAY'S TO-DO LIST:
                                    (A) MUST DO:

AFFIRMATIONS:

VISUALIZATION: (B) WOULD LIKE TO DO:

TODAY'S NOTES:

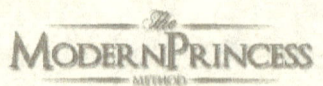

DAILY WEIGHT LOSS DIARY

TODAY'S DATE: _____

NUTRITION LOG:

BREAKFAST:

DINNER:

LUNCH:

SNACKS:

EXERCISE:

FITNESS:

MIND AND SPIRIT:

WAKE UP:

TODAY'S TO-DO LIST:
(A) MUST DO:

AFFIRMATIONS:

VISUALIZATION:

(B) WOULD LIKE TO DO:

TODAY'S NOTES:

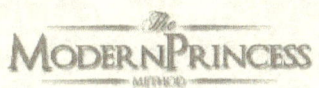

DAILY WEIGHT LOSS DIARY

TODAY'S DATE: _____

NUTRITION LOG:

BREAKFAST:

DINNER:

LUNCH:

SNACKS:

EXERCISE:

FITNESS:

MIND AND SPIRIT:

WAKE UP:

TODAY'S TO-DO LIST:
(A) MUST DO:

AFFIRMATIONS:

VISUALIZATION:

(B) WOULD LIKE TO DO:

TODAY'S NOTES:

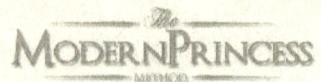

DAILY WEIGHT LOSS DIARY

TODAY'S DATE: _____

NUTRITION LOG:

BREAKFAST: DINNER:

LUNCH: SNACKS:

EXERCISE:

FITNESS:

MIND AND SPIRIT:

WAKE UP: TODAY'S TO-DO LIST:
                                    (A) MUST DO:

AFFIRMATIONS:

VISUALIZATION: (B) WOULD LIKE TO DO:

TODAY'S NOTES:

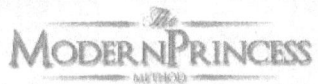

DAILY WEIGHT LOSS DIARY

TODAY'S DATE: _____

NUTRITION LOG:

BREAKFAST:

DINNER:

LUNCH:

SNACKS:

EXERCISE:

FITNESS:

MIND AND SPIRIT:

WAKE UP:

TODAY'S TO-DO LIST:
(A) MUST DO:

AFFIRMATIONS:

VISUALIZATION:

(B) WOULD LIKE TO DO:

TODAY'S NOTES:

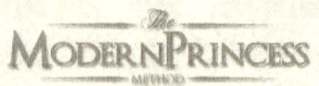

DAILY WEIGHT LOSS DIARY

TODAY'S DATE: _____

NUTRITION LOG:

BREAKFAST: DINNER:

LUNCH: SNACKS:

EXERCISE:

FITNESS:

MIND AND SPIRIT:

WAKE UP: TODAY'S TO-DO LIST:
                                    (A) MUST DO:

AFFIRMATIONS:

VISUALIZATION: (B) WOULD LIKE TO DO:

TODAY'S NOTES:

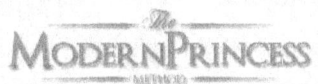

DAILY WEIGHT LOSS DIARY

TODAY'S DATE: _____

NUTRITION LOG:

BREAKFAST:

DINNER:

LUNCH:

SNACKS:

EXERCISE:

FITNESS:

MIND AND SPIRIT:

WAKE UP:

TODAY'S TO-DO LIST:
(A) MUST DO:

AFFIRMATIONS:

VISUALIZATION:

(B) WOULD LIKE TO DO:

TODAY'S NOTES:

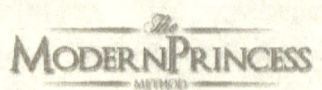

The ModernPrincess
METHOD

DAILY WEIGHT LOSS DIARY

TODAY'S DATE: _____

NUTRITION LOG:

BREAKFAST:

DINNER:

LUNCH:

SNACKS:

EXERCISE:

FITNESS:

MIND AND SPIRIT:

WAKE UP:

TODAY'S TO-DO LIST:
(A) MUST DO:

AFFIRMATIONS:

VISUALIZATION:

(B) WOULD LIKE TO DO:

TODAY'S NOTES:

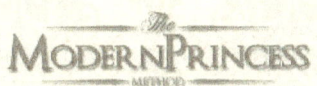

DAILY WEIGHT LOSS DIARY

TODAY'S DATE: _____

NUTRITION LOG:

BREAKFAST: DINNER:

LUNCH: SNACKS:

EXERCISE:

FITNESS:

MIND AND SPIRIT:

WAKE UP: TODAY'S TO-DO LIST:
                                   (A) MUST DO:

AFFIRMATIONS:

VISUALIZATION: (B) WOULD LIKE TO DO:

TODAY'S NOTES:

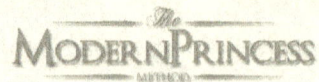

DAILY WEIGHT LOSS DIARY

TODAY'S DATE: _____

NUTRITION LOG:

BREAKFAST:

DINNER:

LUNCH:

SNACKS:

EXERCISE:

FITNESS:

MIND AND SPIRIT:

WAKE UP:

TODAY'S TO-DO LIST:
(A) MUST DO:

AFFIRMATIONS:

VISUALIZATION:

(B) WOULD LIKE TO DO:

TODAY'S NOTES:

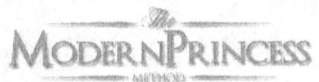

DAILY WEIGHT LOSS DIARY

TODAY'S DATE: _____

NUTRITION LOG:

BREAKFAST:

DINNER:

LUNCH:

SNACKS:

EXERCISE:

FITNESS:

MIND AND SPIRIT:

WAKE UP:

TODAY'S TO-DO LIST:
(A) MUST DO:

AFFIRMATIONS:

VISUALIZATION:

(B) WOULD LIKE TO DO:

TODAY'S NOTES:

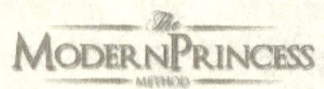

DAILY WEIGHT LOSS DIARY

TODAY'S DATE: _____

NUTRITION LOG:

BREAKFAST:

DINNER:

LUNCH:

SNACKS:

EXERCISE:

FITNESS:

MIND AND SPIRIT:

WAKE UP:

TODAY'S TO-DO LIST:
(A) MUST DO:

AFFIRMATIONS:

VISUALIZATION:

(B) WOULD LIKE TO DO:

TODAY'S NOTES:

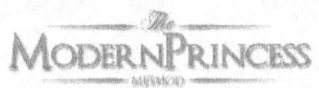

DAILY WEIGHT LOSS DIARY

TODAY'S DATE: _____

NUTRITION LOG:

BREAKFAST:

DINNER:

LUNCH:

SNACKS:

EXERCISE:

FITNESS:

MIND AND SPIRIT:

WAKE UP:

TODAY'S TO-DO LIST:
(A) MUST DO:

AFFIRMATIONS:

VISUALIZATION:

(B) WOULD LIKE TO DO:

TODAY'S NOTES:

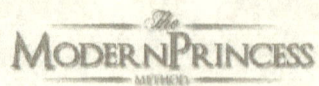

DAILY WEIGHT LOSS DIARY

TODAY'S DATE: _____

NUTRITION LOG:

BREAKFAST:

DINNER:

LUNCH:

SNACKS:

EXERCISE:

FITNESS:

MIND AND SPIRIT:

WAKE UP:

TODAY'S TO-DO LIST:
(A) MUST DO:

AFFIRMATIONS:

VISUALIZATION:

(B) WOULD LIKE TO DO:

TODAY'S NOTES:

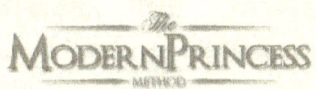
The MODERN PRINCESS METHOD

DAILY WEIGHT LOSS DIARY

TODAY'S DATE: _____

NUTRITION LOG:

BREAKFAST:

DINNER:

LUNCH:

SNACKS:

EXERCISE:

FITNESS:

MIND AND SPIRIT:

WAKE UP:

TODAY'S TO-DO LIST:
(A) MUST DO:

AFFIRMATIONS:

VISUALIZATION:

(B) WOULD LIKE TO DO:

TODAY'S NOTES:

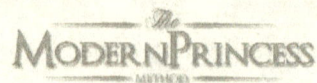

DAILY WEIGHT LOSS DIARY

TODAY'S DATE: _____

NUTRITION LOG:

BREAKFAST:

DINNER:

LUNCH:

SNACKS:

EXERCISE:

FITNESS:

MIND AND SPIRIT:

WAKE UP:

TODAY'S TO-DO LIST:
(A) MUST DO:

AFFIRMATIONS:

VISUALIZATION:

(B) WOULD LIKE TO DO:

TODAY'S NOTES:

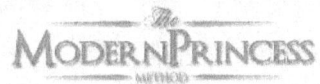

DAILY WEIGHT LOSS DIARY

TODAY'S DATE: _____

NUTRITION LOG:

BREAKFAST:

DINNER:

LUNCH:

SNACKS:

EXERCISE:

FITNESS:

MIND AND SPIRIT:

WAKE UP:

TODAY'S TO-DO LIST:
(A) MUST DO:

AFFIRMATIONS:

VISUALIZATION:

(B) WOULD LIKE TO DO:

TODAY'S NOTES:

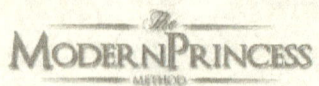
The ModernPrincess
METHOD

DAILY WEIGHT LOSS DIARY

TODAY'S DATE: _____

NUTRITION LOG:

BREAKFAST:

DINNER:

LUNCH:

SNACKS:

EXERCISE:

FITNESS:

MIND AND SPIRIT:

WAKE UP:

TODAY'S TO-DO LIST:
(A) MUST DO:

AFFIRMATIONS:

VISUALIZATION:

(B) WOULD LIKE TO DO:

TODAY'S NOTES:

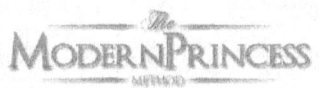

DAILY WEIGHT LOSS DIARY

TODAY'S DATE: _____

NUTRITION LOG:

BREAKFAST:

DINNER:

LUNCH:

SNACKS:

EXERCISE:

FITNESS:

MIND AND SPIRIT:

WAKE UP:

TODAY'S TO-DO LIST:
(A) MUST DO:

AFFIRMATIONS:

VISUALIZATION:

(B) WOULD LIKE TO DO:

TODAY'S NOTES:

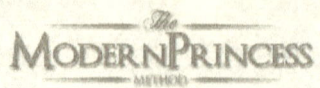

DAILY WEIGHT LOSS DIARY

TODAY'S DATE: _____

NUTRITION LOG:

BREAKFAST:

DINNER:

LUNCH:

SNACKS:

EXERCISE:

FITNESS:

MIND AND SPIRIT:

WAKE UP:

TODAY'S TO-DO LIST:
(A) MUST DO:

AFFIRMATIONS:

VISUALIZATION:

(B) WOULD LIKE TO DO:

TODAY'S NOTES:

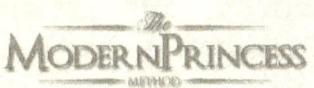

DAILY WEIGHT LOSS DIARY

TODAY'S DATE: _____

NUTRITION LOG:

BREAKFAST:

DINNER:

LUNCH:

SNACKS:

EXERCISE:

FITNESS:

MIND AND SPIRIT:

WAKE UP:

TODAY'S TO-DO LIST:
(A) MUST DO:

AFFIRMATIONS:

VISUALIZATION:

(B) WOULD LIKE TO DO:

TODAY'S NOTES:

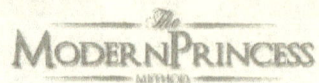
The MODERN PRINCESS
METHOD

DAILY WEIGHT LOSS DIARY

TODAY'S DATE: _____

NUTRITION LOG:

BREAKFAST:

DINNER:

LUNCH:

SNACKS:

EXERCISE:

FITNESS:

MIND AND SPIRIT:

WAKE UP:

TODAY'S TO-DO LIST:
(A) MUST DO:

AFFIRMATIONS:

VISUALIZATION:

(B) WOULD LIKE TO DO:

TODAY'S NOTES:

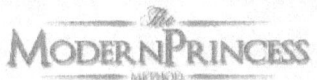

DAILY WEIGHT LOSS DIARY

TODAY'S DATE: _____

NUTRITION LOG:

BREAKFAST:

DINNER:

LUNCH:

SNACKS:

EXERCISE:

FITNESS:

MIND AND SPIRIT:

WAKE UP:

TODAY'S TO-DO LIST:
(A) MUST DO:

AFFIRMATIONS:

VISUALIZATION:

(B) WOULD LIKE TO DO:

TODAY'S NOTES:

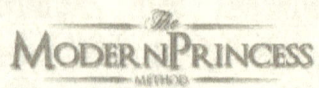
The
MODERNPRINCESS
METHOD

DAILY WEIGHT LOSS DIARY

TODAY'S DATE: _____

NUTRITION LOG:
NUTRITION LOG:

BREAKFAST: DINNER:

LUNCH: SNACKS:

EXERCISE:

FITNESS:

MIND AND SPIRIT:

WAKE UP: TODAY'S TO-DO LIST:
                                    (A) MUST DO:

AFFIRMATIONS:

VISUALIZATION: (B) WOULD LIKE TO DO:

TODAY'S NOTES:

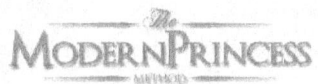

DAILY WEIGHT LOSS DIARY

TODAY'S DATE: _____

NUTRITION LOG:

BREAKFAST:

DINNER:

LUNCH:

SNACKS:

EXERCISE:

FITNESS:

MIND AND SPIRIT:

WAKE UP:

TODAY'S TO-DO LIST:
(A) MUST DO:

AFFIRMATIONS:

VISUALIZATION:

(B) WOULD LIKE TO DO:

TODAY'S NOTES:

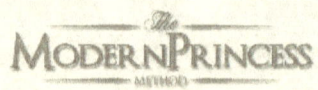

DAILY WEIGHT LOSS DIARY

TODAY'S DATE: _____

NUTRITION LOG:

BREAKFAST: DINNER:

LUNCH: SNACKS:

EXERCISE:

FITNESS:

MIND AND SPIRIT:

WAKE UP: TODAY'S TO-DO LIST:
                                   (A) MUST DO:

AFFIRMATIONS:

VISUALIZATION: (B) WOULD LIKE TO DO:

TODAY'S NOTES:

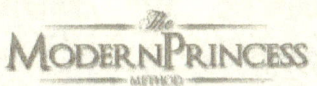

DAILY WEIGHT LOSS DIARY

TODAY'S DATE: _____

NUTRITION LOG:

BREAKFAST:

DINNER:

LUNCH:

SNACKS:

EXERCISE:

FITNESS:

MIND AND SPIRIT:

WAKE UP:

TODAY'S TO-DO LIST:
(A) MUST DO:

AFFIRMATIONS:

VISUALIZATION:

(B) WOULD LIKE TO DO:

TODAY'S NOTES:

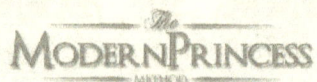

DAILY WEIGHT LOSS DIARY

TODAY'S DATE: _____

NUTRITION LOG:

BREAKFAST:

DINNER:

LUNCH:

SNACKS:

EXERCISE:

FITNESS:

MIND AND SPIRIT:

WAKE UP:

TODAY'S TO-DO LIST:
(A) MUST DO:

AFFIRMATIONS:

VISUALIZATION:

(B) WOULD LIKE TO DO:

TODAY'S NOTES:

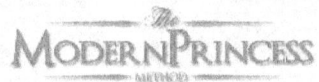

DAILY WEIGHT LOSS DIARY

TODAY'S DATE: _____

NUTRITION LOG:

BREAKFAST:

DINNER:

LUNCH:

SNACKS:

EXERCISE:

FITNESS:

MIND AND SPIRIT:

WAKE UP:

TODAY'S TO-DO LIST:
(A) MUST DO:

AFFIRMATIONS:

VISUALIZATION:

(B) WOULD LIKE TO DO:

TODAY'S NOTES:

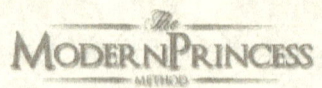
The
MODERNPRINCESS
METHOD

DAILY WEIGHT LOSS DIARY

TODAY'S DATE: _____

NUTRITION LOG:

BREAKFAST: DINNER:

LUNCH: SNACKS:

EXERCISE:

FITNESS:

MIND AND SPIRIT:

WAKE UP: TODAY'S TO-DO LIST:
                                    (A) MUST DO:

AFFIRMATIONS:

VISUALIZATION: (B) WOULD LIKE TO DO:

TODAY'S NOTES:

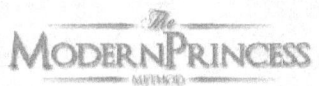

DAILY WEIGHT LOSS DIARY

TODAY'S DATE: _____

NUTRITION LOG:

BREAKFAST: DINNER:

LUNCH: SNACKS:

EXERCISE:

FITNESS:

MIND AND SPIRIT:

WAKE UP: TODAY'S TO-DO LIST:
                                     (A) MUST DO:

AFFIRMATIONS:

VISUALIZATION: (B) WOULD LIKE TO DO:

TODAY'S NOTES:

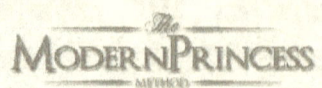

DAILY WEIGHT LOSS DIARY

TODAY'S DATE: _____

NUTRITION LOG:

BREAKFAST:

DINNER:

LUNCH:

SNACKS:

EXERCISE:

FITNESS:

MIND AND SPIRIT:

WAKE UP:

TODAY'S TO-DO LIST:
(A) MUST DO:

AFFIRMATIONS:

VISUALIZATION:

(B) WOULD LIKE TO DO:

TODAY'S NOTES:

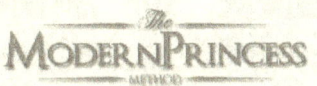

DAILY WEIGHT LOSS DIARY

TODAY'S DATE: _____

NUTRITION LOG:

BREAKFAST:

DINNER:

LUNCH:

SNACKS:

EXERCISE:

FITNESS:

MIND AND SPIRIT:

WAKE UP:

TODAY'S TO-DO LIST:
(A) MUST DO:

AFFIRMATIONS:

VISUALIZATION:

(B) WOULD LIKE TO DO:

TODAY'S NOTES:

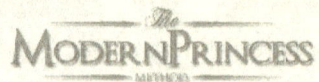

DAILY WEIGHT LOSS DIARY

TODAY'S DATE: _____

NUTRITION LOG:

BREAKFAST:

DINNER:

LUNCH:

SNACKS:

EXERCISE:

FITNESS:

MIND AND SPIRIT:

WAKE UP:

TODAY'S TO-DO LIST:
(A) MUST DO:

AFFIRMATIONS:

VISUALIZATION:

(B) WOULD LIKE TO DO:

TODAY'S NOTES:

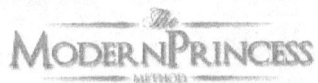

DAILY WEIGHT LOSS DIARY

TODAY'S DATE: _____

NUTRITION LOG:

BREAKFAST:

DINNER:

LUNCH:

SNACKS:

EXERCISE:

FITNESS:

MIND AND SPIRIT:

WAKE UP:

TODAY'S TO-DO LIST:
(A) MUST DO:

AFFIRMATIONS:

VISUALIZATION:

(B) WOULD LIKE TO DO:

TODAY'S NOTES:

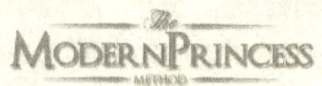

DAILY WEIGHT LOSS DIARY

TODAY'S DATE: _____

NUTRITION LOG:

BREAKFAST:

DINNER:

LUNCH:

SNACKS:

EXERCISE:

FITNESS:

MIND AND SPIRIT:

WAKE UP:

TODAY'S TO-DO LIST:
(A) MUST DO:

AFFIRMATIONS:

VISUALIZATION:

(B) WOULD LIKE TO DO:

TODAY'S NOTES:

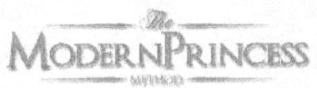

DAILY WEIGHT LOSS DIARY

TODAY'S DATE: _____

NUTRITION LOG:

BREAKFAST:

DINNER:

LUNCH:

SNACKS:

EXERCISE:

FITNESS:

MIND AND SPIRIT:

WAKE UP:

TODAY'S TO-DO LIST:
(A) MUST DO:

AFFIRMATIONS:

VISUALIZATION:

(B) WOULD LIKE TO DO:

TODAY'S NOTES:

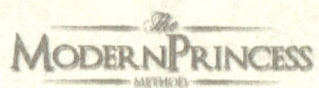

DAILY WEIGHT LOSS DIARY

TODAY'S DATE: _____

NUTRITION LOG:

BREAKFAST:

DINNER:

LUNCH:

SNACKS:

EXERCISE:

FITNESS:

MIND AND SPIRIT:

WAKE UP:

TODAY'S TO-DO LIST:
(A) MUST DO:

AFFIRMATIONS:

VISUALIZATION:

(B) WOULD LIKE TO DO:

TODAY'S NOTES:

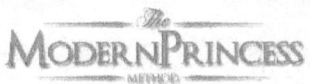

DAILY WEIGHT LOSS DIARY

TODAY'S DATE: _____

NUTRITION LOG:

BREAKFAST: DINNER:

LUNCH: SNACKS:

EXERCISE:

FITNESS:

MIND AND SPIRIT:

WAKE UP: TODAY'S TO-DO LIST:
                                    (A) MUST DO:

AFFIRMATIONS:

VISUALIZATION: (B) WOULD LIKE TO DO:

TODAY'S NOTES:

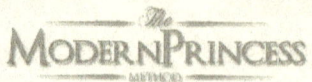

DAILY WEIGHT LOSS DIARY

TODAY'S DATE: _____

NUTRITION LOG:

BREAKFAST:

DINNER:

LUNCH:

SNACKS:

EXERCISE:

FITNESS:

MIND AND SPIRIT:

WAKE UP:

TODAY'S TO-DO LIST:
(A) MUST DO:

AFFIRMATIONS:

VISUALIZATION:

(B) WOULD LIKE TO DO:

TODAY'S NOTES:

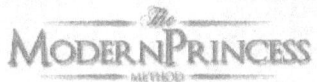

DAILY WEIGHT LOSS DIARY

TODAY'S DATE: _____

NUTRITION LOG:

BREAKFAST:

DINNER:

LUNCH:

SNACKS:

EXERCISE:

FITNESS:

MIND AND SPIRIT:

WAKE UP:

TODAY'S TO-DO LIST:
(A) MUST DO:

AFFIRMATIONS:

VISUALIZATION:

(B) WOULD LIKE TO DO:

TODAY'S NOTES:

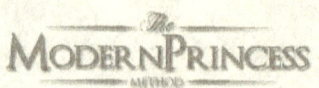

DAILY WEIGHT LOSS DIARY

TODAY'S DATE: _____

NUTRITION LOG:

BREAKFAST:

DINNER:

LUNCH:

SNACKS:

EXERCISE:

FITNESS:

MIND AND SPIRIT:

WAKE UP:

TODAY'S TO-DO LIST:
(A) MUST DO:

AFFIRMATIONS:

VISUALIZATION:

(B) WOULD LIKE TO DO:

TODAY'S NOTES:

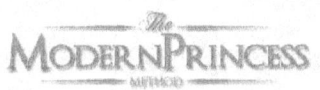

DAILY WEIGHT LOSS DIARY

TODAY'S DATE: _____

NUTRITION LOG:

BREAKFAST:

DINNER:

LUNCH:

SNACKS:

EXERCISE:

FITNESS:

MIND AND SPIRIT:

WAKE UP:

TODAY'S TO-DO LIST:
(A) MUST DO:

AFFIRMATIONS:

VISUALIZATION:

(B) WOULD LIKE TO DO:

TODAY'S NOTES:

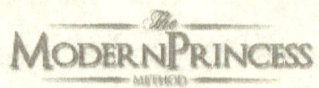

DAILY WEIGHT LOSS DIARY

TODAY'S DATE: _____

NUTRITION LOG:

BREAKFAST:

DINNER:

LUNCH:

SNACKS:

EXERCISE:

FITNESS:

MIND AND SPIRIT:

WAKE UP:

TODAY'S TO-DO LIST:
(A) MUST DO:

AFFIRMATIONS:

VISUALIZATION:

(B) WOULD LIKE TO DO:

TODAY'S NOTES:

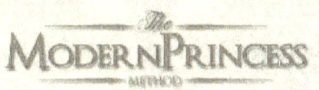

DAILY WEIGHT LOSS DIARY

TODAY'S DATE: _____

NUTRITION LOG:

BREAKFAST: DINNER:

LUNCH: SNACKS:

EXERCISE:

FITNESS:

MIND AND SPIRIT:

WAKE UP: TODAY'S TO-DO LIST:
                                  (A) MUST DO:

AFFIRMATIONS:

VISUALIZATION: (B) WOULD LIKE TO DO:

TODAY'S NOTES:

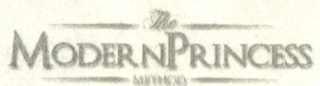

DAILY WEIGHT LOSS DIARY

TODAY'S DATE: _____

NUTRITION LOG:

BREAKFAST:

DINNER:

LUNCH:

SNACKS:

EXERCISE:

FITNESS:

MIND AND SPIRIT:

WAKE UP:

TODAY'S TO-DO LIST:
(A) MUST DO:

AFFIRMATIONS:

VISUALIZATION:

(B) WOULD LIKE TO DO:

TODAY'S NOTES:

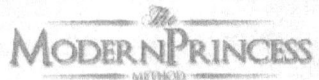

DAILY WEIGHT LOSS DIARY

TODAY'S DATE: _____

NUTRITION LOG:

BREAKFAST:

DINNER:

LUNCH:

SNACKS:

EXERCISE:

FITNESS:

MIND AND SPIRIT:

WAKE UP:

TODAY'S TO-DO LIST:
(A) MUST DO:

AFFIRMATIONS:

VISUALIZATION:

(B) WOULD LIKE TO DO:

TODAY'S NOTES:

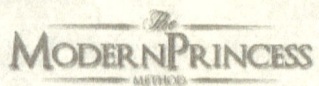

DAILY WEIGHT LOSS DIARY

TODAY'S DATE: _____

NUTRITION LOG:

BREAKFAST:

DINNER:

LUNCH:

SNACKS:

EXERCISE:

FITNESS:

MIND AND SPIRIT:

WAKE UP:

TODAY'S TO-DO LIST:
(A) MUST DO:

AFFIRMATIONS:

VISUALIZATION:

(B) WOULD LIKE TO DO:

TODAY'S NOTES:

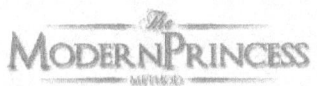

DAILY WEIGHT LOSS DIARY

TODAY'S DATE: _____

NUTRITION LOG:

BREAKFAST:

DINNER:

LUNCH:

SNACKS:

EXERCISE:

FITNESS:

MIND AND SPIRIT:

WAKE UP:

TODAY'S TO-DO LIST:
(A) MUST DO:

AFFIRMATIONS:

VISUALIZATION:

(B) WOULD LIKE TO DO:

TODAY'S NOTES:

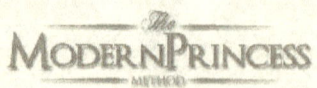

DAILY WEIGHT LOSS DIARY

TODAY'S DATE: _____

NUTRITION LOG:

BREAKFAST:

DINNER:

LUNCH:

SNACKS:

EXERCISE:

FITNESS:

MIND AND SPIRIT:

WAKE UP:

TODAY'S TO-DO LIST:
(A) MUST DO:

AFFIRMATIONS:

VISUALIZATION:

(B) WOULD LIKE TO DO:

TODAY'S NOTES:

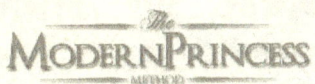

DAILY WEIGHT LOSS DIARY

TODAY'S DATE: _____

NUTRITION LOG:

BREAKFAST:

DINNER:

LUNCH:

SNACKS:

EXERCISE:

FITNESS:

MIND AND SPIRIT:

WAKE UP:

TODAY'S TO-DO LIST:
(A) MUST DO:

AFFIRMATIONS:

VISUALIZATION:

(B) WOULD LIKE TO DO:

TODAY'S NOTES:

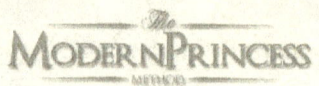

DAILY WEIGHT LOSS DIARY

TODAY'S DATE: _____

NUTRITION LOG:

BREAKFAST:

DINNER:

LUNCH:

SNACKS:

EXERCISE:

FITNESS:

MIND AND SPIRIT:

WAKE UP:

TODAY'S TO-DO LIST:
(A) MUST DO:

AFFIRMATIONS:

VISUALIZATION:

(B) WOULD LIKE TO DO:

TODAY'S NOTES:

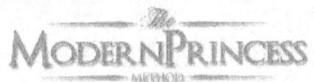

DAILY WEIGHT LOSS DIARY

TODAY'S DATE: _____

NUTRITION LOG:

BREAKFAST:

DINNER:

LUNCH:

SNACKS:

EXERCISE:

FITNESS:

MIND AND SPIRIT:

WAKE UP:

TODAY'S TO-DO LIST:
(A) MUST DO:

AFFIRMATIONS:

VISUALIZATION:

(B) WOULD LIKE TO DO:

TODAY'S NOTES:

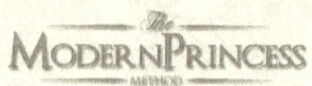

DAILY WEIGHT LOSS DIARY

TODAY'S DATE: _____

NUTRITION LOG:

BREAKFAST:

DINNER:

LUNCH:

SNACKS:

EXERCISE:

FITNESS:

MIND AND SPIRIT:

WAKE UP:

TODAY'S TO-DO LIST:
(A) MUST DO:

AFFIRMATIONS:

VISUALIZATION:

(B) WOULD LIKE TO DO:

TODAY'S NOTES:

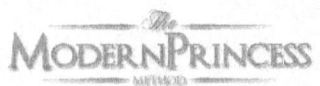

DAILY WEIGHT LOSS DIARY

TODAY'S DATE: _____

NUTRITION LOG:

BREAKFAST:

DINNER:

LUNCH:

SNACKS:

EXERCISE:

FITNESS:

MIND AND SPIRIT:

WAKE UP:

TODAY'S TO-DO LIST:
(A) MUST DO:

AFFIRMATIONS:

VISUALIZATION:

(B) WOULD LIKE TO DO:

TODAY'S NOTES:

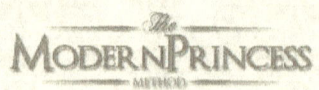

DAILY WEIGHT LOSS DIARY

TODAY'S DATE: _____

NUTRITION LOG:

BREAKFAST:

DINNER:

LUNCH:

SNACKS:

EXERCISE:

FITNESS:

MIND AND SPIRIT:

WAKE UP:

TODAY'S TO-DO LIST:
(A) MUST DO:

AFFIRMATIONS:

VISUALIZATION:

(B) WOULD LIKE TO DO:

TODAY'S NOTES:

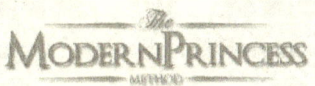

DAILY WEIGHT LOSS DIARY

TODAY'S DATE: _____

NUTRITION LOG:

BREAKFAST:

DINNER:

LUNCH:

SNACKS:

EXERCISE:

FITNESS:

MIND AND SPIRIT:

WAKE UP:

TODAY'S TO-DO LIST:
(A) MUST DO:

AFFIRMATIONS:

VISUALIZATION:

(B) WOULD LIKE TO DO:

TODAY'S NOTES:

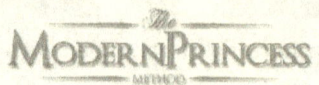

DAILY WEIGHT LOSS DIARY

TODAY'S DATE: _____

NUTRITION LOG:

BREAKFAST: DINNER:

LUNCH: SNACKS:

EXERCISE:

FITNESS:

MIND AND SPIRIT:

WAKE UP: TODAY'S TO-DO LIST:
                                   (A) MUST DO:

AFFIRMATIONS:

VISUALIZATION: (B) WOULD LIKE TO DO:

TODAY'S NOTES:

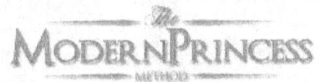

DAILY WEIGHT LOSS DIARY

TODAY'S DATE: _____

NUTRITION LOG:

BREAKFAST: DINNER:

LUNCH: SNACKS:

EXERCISE:

FITNESS:

MIND AND SPIRIT:

WAKE UP: TODAY'S TO-DO LIST:
                                    (A) MUST DO:

AFFIRMATIONS:

VISUALIZATION: (B) WOULD LIKE TO DO:

TODAY'S NOTES:

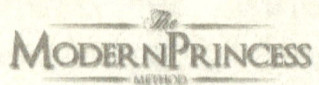

DAILY WEIGHT LOSS DIARY

TODAY'S DATE: _____

NUTRITION LOG:

BREAKFAST: DINNER:

LUNCH: SNACKS:

EXERCISE:

FITNESS:

MIND AND SPIRIT:

WAKE UP: TODAY'S TO-DO LIST:
                                        (A) MUST DO:

AFFIRMATIONS:

VISUALIZATION: (B) WOULD LIKE TO DO:

TODAY'S NOTES:

www.ingramcontent.com/pod-product-compliance
Lightning Source LLC
Chambersburg PA
CBHW020357290526
45785CB00005B/2335